THE AGELESS MIND RECIPES

The Ultimate Guide to Anti-Aging Rituals

MOH LIMS

ACKNOWLEDGEMENT

We extend our heartfelt gratitude to all those who made this endeavor possible.

Our deepest appreciation goes to the dedicated team of researchers, culinary experts, and health professionals whose tireless efforts brought these The Ageless Mind Recipes to fruition.

We also thank our cherished readers for embarking on this transformative journey with us. Your passion for self-care and pursuit of well-being fuel our commitment to provide valuable resources.

Together, we embrace the wisdom of the ages and step confidently into a future where vitality and grace know no boundaries.

DEDUCTION

In the grand tapestry of life, the pursuit of youthfulness and longevity is a timeless endeavor.

Through the exploration of **The Ageless Mind Recipes**, we have harnessed the power of nature's bounties, blending culinary art with scientific wisdom. These recipes, carefully curated to nourish both body and soul, offer a glimpse of the extraordinary possibilities that lie within our grasp.

As we close this chapter, let us carry forth the knowledge and practices gained, forever empowered to savor the richness of life and bask in the brilliance of our ageless essence.

TABLE OF CONTENT

INTRODUCTION

In the relentless march of time, humanity has long sought the elusive secret to halting its relentless effects on our bodies and minds.

The quest for eternal youth and vitality has spanned generations, transcending cultures, and driving us to uncover the hidden elixirs of life. Welcome to a world where science, nature, and culinary art converge to offer a potent solution - a collection of The Ageless Mind Recipes.

As we embark on this journey, we will explore a treasure trove of nourishing ingredients, masterfully blended to not only tantalize the taste buds but also to rejuvenate and revitalize from within.

These recipes are not merely culinary creations; they are a celebration of life and a testament to the human spirit's unyielding pursuit of longevity and well-being.

Within the chapters that follow, you will discover an array of delightful smoothies and juices, brimming with antioxidants and vitamins to combat the ravages of time. You will savor sumptuous salads, vibrant with colors and flavors, enhancing your skin's radiance and promoting youthful elasticity.

Prepare to indulge in main courses that nourish both body and soul, featuring superfoods that protect and fortify your very essence. As we venture into the realm of desserts, you will find that satisfying your sweet tooth can also be a path to ageless allure, with dark chocolates and berries providing potent allies in the fight against premature aging.

But our quest does not end there. From invigorating beverages to face masks, body scrubs, and luxurious serums, we have curated an arsenal of natural remedies and self-care rituals to defy the hands of time.

Each chapter unlocks the potential of ingredients that mother nature has bestowed upon us, showcasing the wonders they hold in their embrace.

So, take a leap into the world of The Ageless Mind Recipes, where each bite and sip, each touch and application, are a harmonious symphony orchestrating the dance of youth and vitality.

Embrace this culinary odyssey with an open heart and a willing spirit, for within these pages lies the potential to unlock a timeless secret - the key to a more vibrant, healthier, and ageless you.

Smoothies And Juices

1. Anti-Aging Berry Blast Smoothie

Ingredients:

- 1 cup mixed berries (blueberries, strawberries, raspberries)
- 1 banana
- 1/2 cup Greek yogurt
- 1 tablespoon chia seeds
- 1 cup spinach
- 1 cup almond milk

Instructions:

1. Add all the ingredients to a blender.
2. Blend until smooth and creamy.
3. Pour into a glass and enjoy!

Benefits:

- Rich in antioxidants to combat free radicals.
- The vitamins in berries promote collagen production for youthful skin.

2. Green Anti-Aging Juice

Ingredients:

- 2 cucumbers
- 2 green apples
- 2 cups kale
- 1 lemon
- 1-inch piece of ginger

Instructions:

1. Wash and chop all the ingredients.
2. Pass them through a juicer.
3. Stir well and serve immediately.

Benefits:

- High in chlorophyll, aiding in detoxification and reducing skin inflammation.
- Vitamin C from the lemon boosts skin radiance.

Salads

3. Avocado and Tomato Salad

Ingredients:

- 2 ripe avocados, diced

- 2 cups cherry tomatoes, halved

- 1/4 cup red onion, finely chopped

- 2 tablespoons extra-virgin olive oil

- 1 tablespoon balsamic vinegar

- Salt and pepper to taste

Instructions:

1. In a large bowl, combine avocados, tomatoes, and red onion.

2. Drizzle with olive oil and balsamic vinegar.

3. Season with salt and pepper, then toss gently to combine.

Benefits:

- Avocado provides healthy fats and vitamin E for skin nourishment.

- Tomatoes contain lycopene, known to protect against sun damage.

4. Quinoa and Kale Salad

Ingredients:

- 1 cup cooked quinoa
- 2 cups chopped kale
- 1/2 cup pomegranate seeds
- 1/4 cup feta cheese, crumbled
- 1/4 cup toasted almonds
- 2 tablespoons olive oil
- 1 tablespoon lemon juice
- Salt and pepper to taste

Instructions:

1. In a large bowl, mix quinoa, kale, pomegranate seeds, feta cheese, and almonds.
2. In a separate bowl, whisk together olive oil, lemon juice, salt, and pepper.
3. Pour the dressing over the salad and toss gently.

Benefits:

- Quinoa is rich in protein and amino acids for collagen production.
- Kale is packed with vitamins A, C, and K, promoting skin elasticity.

Main Courses

5. Grilled Salmon with Lemon-Dill Sauce

Ingredients:

- 4 salmon fillets
- 2 lemons
- 2 tablespoons fresh dill, chopped
- 1 tablespoon olive oil
- Salt and pepper to taste

Instructions:

1. Preheat the grill or oven to medium-high heat.
2. Season the salmon fillets with salt and pepper.
3. Grill or bake the salmon until cooked through.
4. In a small bowl, mix the juice of one lemon with dill and olive oil.
5. Drizzle the lemon-dill sauce over the cooked salmon and serve with lemon slices.

Benefits:

- Salmon is rich in omega-3 fatty acids, supporting skin hydration.
- Lemon and dill add antioxidants for skin health.

6. Tofu Stir-Fry with Broccoli and Ginger

Ingredients:

- 1 block firm tofu, cubed

- 2 cups broccoli florets

- 1 red bell pepper, sliced

- 2 tablespoons soy sauce

- 1 tablespoon sesame oil

- 1 tablespoon fresh ginger, minced

- 2 cloves garlic, minced

- 2 green onions, chopped

- Sesame seeds for garnish

Instructions:

1. In a large skillet, heat sesame oil over medium heat.

2. Add tofu and stir-fry until golden brown.

3. Add broccoli, bell pepper, ginger, and garlic. Cook for a few minutes until veggies are tender-crisp.

4. Stir in soy sauce and green onions. Cook for another minute.

5. Garnish with sesame seeds before serving.

Benefits:

- Tofu provides plant-based protein and helps reduce the breakdown of collagen.

- Ginger contains anti-inflammatory properties beneficial for the skin.

Desserts

7. Dark Chocolate and Mixed Berries Parfait

Ingredients:

- 1 cup Greek yogurt

- 1 tablespoon honey

- 1/4 cup dark chocolate chips

- 1 cup mixed berries (blueberries, strawberries, raspberries)

- 1/4 cup granola

Instructions:

1. In a bowl, mix Greek yogurt and honey until well combined.

2. Layer the yogurt mixture, dark chocolate chips, mixed berries, and granola in a glass.

3. Repeat the layers until the glass is filled.

Benefits:

- Dark chocolate is rich in flavonoids, promoting skin hydration and elasticity.

- Berries offer a range of antioxidants for youthful skin.

8. Chia Seed Pudding

Ingredients:

- 1/4 cup chia seeds
- 1 cup almond milk
- 1 tablespoon maple syrup
- 1/2 teaspoon vanilla extract
- Sliced fruits (e.g., mango, kiwi, berries) for topping

Instructions:

1. In a bowl, mix chia seeds, almond milk, maple syrup, and vanilla extract.
2. Stir well and let it sit for at least 2 hours or overnight in the refrigerator.
3. Before serving, top with sliced fruits.

Benefits:

- Chia seeds are packed with omega-3 fatty acids and antioxidants.
- Almond milk offers vitamin E and healthy fats for skin nourishment.

Snacks

9. Kale Chips

Ingredients:

- 1 bunch kale, washed and dried

- 1 tablespoon olive oil

- 1/2 teaspoon sea salt

- 1/2 teaspoon garlic powder

Instructions:

1. Preheat the oven to 350°F (175°C).

2. Remove the tough stems from the kale leaves and tear them into bite-sized pieces.

3. In a large bowl, toss the kale with olive oil, sea salt, and garlic powder.

4. Spread the kale on a baking sheet in a single layer.

5. Bake for 10-15 minutes until crispy.

Benefits:

- Kale is an excellent source of vitamin A, C, and K, promoting skin health.

- Olive oil provides healthy fats for moisturized skin.

10. Almond and Date Energy Bites

Ingredients:

- 1 cup almonds
- 1 cup pitted dates
- 1 tablespoon almond butter
- 1 tablespoon cocoa powder
- 1/2 teaspoon vanilla extract
- Shredded coconut for coating

Instructions:

1. In a food processor, blend almonds until finely ground.

2. Add dates, almond butter, cocoa powder, and vanilla extract. Blend until a sticky mixture forms.

3. Roll the mixture into small balls and coat them with shredded coconut.

Benefits:

- Almonds are a source of vitamin E and antioxidants.
- Dates offer natural sweetness and fiber for healthy digestion.

Beverages

11. Green Tea with Lemon and Honey

Ingredients:

- 2 green tea bags

- 2 cups hot water

- Juice of half a lemon

- 1 tablespoon honey

Instructions:

1. Steep the green tea bags in hot water for 3-4 minutes.

2. Remove the tea bags and add lemon juice and honey.

3. Stir until the honey dissolves.

4. Serve warm or over ice.

Benefits:

- Green tea contains polyphenols that protect against skin aging.

- Lemon provides vitamin C and enhances skin radiance.

12.   Golden Milk Latte

Ingredients:

- 1 cup unsweetened almond milk
- 1 teaspoon turmeric powder
- 1/2 teaspoon cinnamon
- 1/4 teaspoon ground ginger
- 1 tablespoon honey or maple syrup
- Pinch of black pepper

Instructions:

1. In a small saucepan, heat almond milk over medium heat.

2. Whisk in turmeric, cinnamon, ginger, honey or maple syrup, and black pepper.

3. Heat until warm, but not boiling.

4. Pour into a cup and sprinkle with a pinch of cinnamon.

Benefits:

- Turmeric has anti-inflammatory and antioxidant properties for youthful skin.
- Cinnamon helps regulate blood sugar levels, supporting overall health.

Face Masks

13. Nourishing Avocado Face Mask

Ingredients:

- 1 ripe avocado, mashed
- 1 tablespoon honey
- 1 tablespoon plain yogurt
- 1 teaspoon olive oil

Instructions:

1. In a bowl, mix mashed avocado, honey, yogurt, and olive oil until smooth.
2. Apply the mask to your face and neck, avoiding the eye area.
3. Leave it on for 15-20 minutes, then rinse off with warm water.

Benefits:

- Avocado nourishes the skin with healthy fats and vitamins.
- Honey and yogurt soothe and moisturize the skin.

14. Brightening Turmeric Face Mask

Ingredients:

- 1 tablespoon turmeric powder

- 1 tablespoon yogurt

- 1 teaspoon honey

Instructions:

1. In a bowl, mix turmeric powder, yogurt, and honey until well combined.

2. Apply the mask to your face and leave it on for 10-15 minutes.

3. Rinse off with warm water, gently massaging the skin in circular motions.

Benefits:

- Turmeric brightens the skin and reduces dark spots.

- Yogurt and honey provide hydration and a youthful glow.

Body Scrubs

15.   Coconut and Brown Sugar Scrub

Ingredients:

- 1/2 cup coconut oil

- 1 cup brown sugar

- 1 teaspoon vanilla extract

Instructions:

1. In a bowl, mix coconut oil, brown sugar, and vanilla extract until combined.

2. Gently massage the scrub onto damp skin in circular motions.

3. Rinse off with warm water.

Benefits:

- Coconut oil moisturizes and softens the skin.

- Brown sugar exfoliates and removes dead skin cells.

16.   Coffee and Cocoa Body Scrub

Ingredients:

- 1/2 cup coffee grounds

- 1/2 cup cocoa powder

- 1/4 cup coconut oil

- 1 tablespoon honey

Instructions:

1. In a bowl, mix coffee grounds, cocoa powder, coconut oil, and honey.

2. Apply the scrub to wet skin and massage gently.

3. Rinse off thoroughly with warm water.

Benefits:

- Coffee stimulates blood flow and reduces the appearance of cellulite.

- Cocoa powder is rich in antioxidants, promoting skin repair.

Face Serums

17.　Hydrating Rosehip Seed Oil Serum

Ingredients:

- 2 tablespoons rosehip seed oil
- 5 drops vitamin E oil
- 3 drops lavender essential oil

Instructions:

1. In a small dropper bottle, combine rosehip seed oil, vitamin E oil, and lavender essential oil.
2. Shake well before use.
3. Apply a few drops to clean, damp skin and gently massage in upward motions.

Benefits:

- Rosehip seed oil is rich in essential fatty acids and vitamin A, reducing wrinkles and fine lines.
- Lavender essential oil calms and soothes the skin.

18.　Rejuvenating Frankincense Serum

Ingredients:

- 2 tablespoons argan oil
- 5 drops frankincense essential oil

- 3 drops geranium essential oil

Instructions:

1. In a small dropper bottle, combine argan oil, frankincense essential oil, and geranium essential oil.

2. Shake well before use.

3. Apply a few drops to clean, damp skin and massage gently.

Benefits:

- Argan oil provides moisture and nourishment for mature skin.

- Frankincense and geranium essential oils promote cell regeneration.

Body Lotions

19. Shea Butter and Lavender Body Lotion

Ingredients:

- 1/2 cup shea butter

- 1/4 cup coconut oil

- 1 tablespoon almond oil

- 10 drops lavender essential oil

Instructions:

1. In a double boiler, melt shea butter and coconut oil together.

2. Remove from heat and let it cool for a few minutes.

3. Stir in almond oil and lavender essential oil.

4. Transfer the mixture to a jar and let it solidify.

Benefits:

- Shea butter is deeply moisturizing and nourishing for the skin.

- Lavender essential oil has calming properties, aiding relaxation.

20. Aloe Vera and Calendula Body Lotion

Ingredients:

- 1/2 cup aloe vera gel

- 1/4 cup almond oil

- 1 tablespoon beeswax pellets

- 1 tablespoon calendula oil

- 10 drops chamomile essential oil

Instructions:

1. In a double boiler, melt beeswax pellets and almond oil together.

2. Remove from heat and let it cool slightly.

3. Stir in aloe vera gel, calendula oil, and chamomile essential oil.

4. Transfer the lotion to a container and let it set.

Benefits:

- Aloe vera soothes and hydrates the skin, reducing redness.

- Calendula and chamomile oils have anti-inflammatory properties for sensitive skin.

CONCLUSION

As we reach the culmination of our The Ageless Mind Recipes journey, we stand at the precipice of newfound knowledge and empowerment. The pages of this collection have illuminated the path to preserving youthfulness and embracing a lifestyle that celebrates vitality.

By incorporating these nourishing recipes and self-care rituals into our lives, we have armed ourselves with potent tools to combat the sands of time.

Let us remember that the pursuit of anti-aging extends far beyond the confines of vanity. It is an ode to self-love, an acknowledgment of the temple we inhabit, and a commitment to cherishing the gift of life.

As we savor the flavors, textures, and benefits that each recipe bestows, let us savor the joy of nurturing ourselves holistically.

To the astute buyer of this treasure trove, we extend our heartfelt appreciation for your trust and dedication to the practice of self-care.

Your journey towards ageless allure is a testament to your unwavering commitment to well-being and the beauty that radiates from within.

May these recipes continue to be your companions in the quest for timeless elegance and may they bring you boundless joy, health, and rejuvenation.

Congratulations on embracing this transformative adventure, and may your path be forever aglow with the radiance of eternal youth.